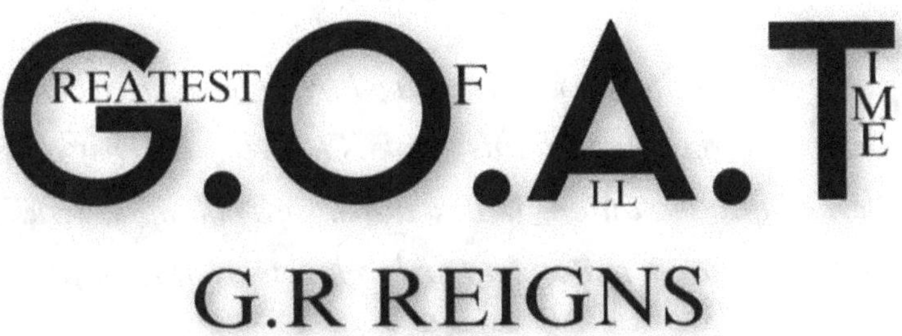

Greatest of All Time: Achieving the Legendary Status

GRAYSON REIGNS

PUBLISHER

BookJet Publicity

New York, NY

Dedication

To all the men out there who are struggling to navigate what it means to be a man in today's world, this book is for you. It's easy to feel like you're being pulled in different directions, with changing gender roles and societal pressures making it hard to know what masculinity even means anymore.

But I want you to know that it's possible to be a strong, powerful man in today's world, no matter what anyone else might say. You define your own masculinity, and you have the power to shape it in a way that feels authentic and true to you.

It's not always easy to cultivate that inner strength and resilience that makes a man truly powerful. It takes hard work, dedication, and a willingness to confront your fears and weaknesses head-on. But I want you to know that it's worth it. When you have that inner strength, that unshakable sense of purpose, you become unstoppable.

So I invite you to read this book with an open mind and an open heart. Take what resonates with you, leave what doesn't, and above all, remember that you have the power to shape your own destiny and become the best version of yourself.

Here's to all the men out there who are willing to put in the work, to face their fears and weaknesses head-on, and to become the strong, powerful men they were meant to be. Let's do this!

Table of Contents

PENMAN'S NOTE

Alright fellas, listen up. I know some of you are feeling like the world is trying to emasculate you, make you weak and compliant. But let me tell you something: you don't have to let it. You can still be a powerful, dominant man in today's world, but you have to be willing to put in the work.

First off, forget about what anyone else says about what it means to be a man. You define that for yourself.

You want to be emotional? **Fine.**

You want to be stoic and tough? **Fine.**

But whatever you choose, **own it.**

Don't let anyone else tell you how to live your life.

Now, cultivating inner strength and resilience is no easy task. It takes discipline, dedication, and a willingness to face your fears head-on. But let me tell you, the rewards are worth it. When you have that inner strength, that unshakable sense of purpose, you become unstoppable. You can handle whatever life throws your way and come out on top.

So here's what you need to do. First, figure out what you want in life. What are your goals? What drives you? Once you have that, make a plan and start taking action. No excuses, no half-measures. You have to be all in.

Second, don't be afraid to seek out mentors and resources that can help you along the way. Whether it's a coach, a book, or a community of like-minded individuals, find something that will keep you accountable and help you grow.

Finally, never stop pushing yourself. Don't settle for mediocrity or complacency. Always be striving for excellence. That's what being a man is all about: pushing yourself to be the best you can be.

So don't let anyone else define your masculinity. You define it for yourself. And if you're willing to put in the work, you can be a powerful, dominant force in today's world.

Are you ready, soldier?

Alright fellas, listen up. If you want to be a real man, you need to finish this book, adapt what you learn to your own life, and apply it every damn day. Because let me tell you something: the world is getting tougher, and we need to be stronger to protect ourselves and the people we love.

Now, I know some of you might be hesitant. You might be thinking, "I don't know if I'm ready for this kind of change." Well, if that's the case, then do yourself a favor and give this book to someone who is ready. Someone who is willing to stand up and rip those chains of weakness off themselves, to become the strong, powerful men they were meant to be.

But if you are ready, then I promise you, this book can be a game-changer. It can give you the tools you need to cultivate inner strength, resilience, and purpose. It can help you define your own masculinity, on your own terms, without letting anyone else tell you who you should be.

But the key is that you have to be willing to put in the work. You can't just read this book and expect everything to magically change. You have to take what you learn, and apply it in your daily life. You have to be willing to face your fears, confront your weaknesses, and push yourself to be better every day.

So if you're ready for that kind of change, then let's do this. Let's read this book together, and let's become the strong, powerful men that we were meant to be.

G.O.A.T

Greatest of All Time: Achieving the Legendary Status

G.O.A.T Rule #1 | F**k the Haters: Embracing Your Inner Alpha

> *In a world of sheep, be a f*cking lion. Embrace your power and show the world what you're capable of.*

Alright, let's get real. The G.O.A.T Rule #1 is all about embracing your inner alpha and showing the world what you're made of.

The first rule? F**k the haters.

That's right, you heard me. Don't let anyone else's opinions or doubts bring you down. You are the captain of your own ship, and you get to decide where it sails. So, throw up a middle finger to anyone who tries to tear you down, and embrace your inner strength.

But embracing your inner alpha isn't just about giving a big "F you" to the world. It's also about taking action and living life on your own terms. That means setting goals, making plans, and following through with them, no matter what anyone else says. It means being confident in your decisions, and not second-guessing yourself. It means taking risks and being willing to fail, because you know that's the only way to truly succeed.

So, how do you embrace your inner alpha? First, start by identifying what makes you feel strong and confident. Maybe it's hitting the gym and pushing yourself to new limits. Maybe it's taking on a new challenge at work, or pursuing a passion project that you've been putting off. Whatever it is, make it a priority in your life, and commit to it fully.

Next, surround yourself with people who lift you up and support you. You don't need negative energy in your life, so cut ties with anyone who tries to hold you back or bring you down. Instead, seek out friends and mentors who share your values and push you to be your best self.

Finally, don't be afraid to take up space and be bold. Stand up straight, make eye contact, and speak your mind. Embrace your strengths and acknowledge your weaknesses, but never apologize for who you are. Remember, you are a warrior, and warriors don't back down from a challenge. So, go out there and conquer the world, on your own terms. That's the true Warriors Code.

Another important aspect of embracing your inner alpha is taking ownership of your life. Don't make excuses or blame others for your problems. Take responsibility for your actions and decisions, and learn from your mistakes. This doesn't mean that you have to be perfect, but it does mean that you have to be accountable.

In addition, learn to cultivate a mindset of abundance rather than scarcity. Don't compare yourself to others or get caught up in jealousy or envy. Instead, focus on your own journey and celebrate your successes, no matter how small they may seem. Remember, there is enough success and happiness to go around for everyone, and there's no need to tear others down in order to build yourself up.

Another key part of the G.O.A.T Rule #1 is staying true to your values and beliefs. Don't compromise your integrity or morals in order to fit in or please others. Stand up for what you believe in, even if it's not popular or easy. This doesn't mean that you should be closed-minded or unwilling to listen to others, but it does mean that you should have the courage to speak up when you see injustice or wrongdoing.

Finally, it's important to stay humble and grounded as you embrace your inner alpha. Don't let your success or confidence go to your head. Remember that there is always more to learn and room to grow, and that true strength comes from a place of humility and gratitude.

In conclusion, the G.O.A.T Rule #1 is about embracing your inner strength, confidence, and leadership. It's about taking ownership of your life, staying true to your values, and living with courage and integrity. So, go forth and embrace your inner alpha, and show the world what you're made of. The world needs more warriors like you.

To truly embrace your inner alpha, it's important to work on developing a strong and confident mindset. This means focusing on positive self-talk, visualizing success, and cultivating a sense of resilience in the face of setbacks or challenges.

One way to do this is by setting goals and breaking them down into manageable steps. By focusing on small wins and progress, you'll build momentum and confidence over time. You can also try practicing mindfulness and meditation to help calm your mind and stay centered in the present moment.

Another important part of the G.O.A.T Rule #1 is building strong relationships and connections with others. This means learning to communicate effectively, listen actively, and show empathy and compassion. When you can connect with others on a deeper level, you'll be better equipped to build trust, resolve conflicts, and achieve common goals.

It's also important to take care of your physical health, as this can have a big impact on your mental and emotional well-being. This means getting enough sleep, eating a healthy and balanced diet, and staying active through regular exercise. When you feel strong and healthy, you'll have more energy and focus to tackle your goals and challenges.

In the end, embracing your inner alpha is about being true to yourself, owning your strengths and weaknesses, and living with courage and integrity. By following the Warriors Code, you can build a life that is fulfilling, meaningful, and full of purpose. So, go forth and show the world what you're made of. The world needs more warriors like you.

G.O.A.T Rule #2 | Unbreakable Mental Resilience: Developing the Iron Will

> *"*
>
> *Being a true champion requires the ability to weather any storm - the strongest steel is forged in the hottest fires, and the same is true for your mental resilience.*

Listen up, soldiers. In this world, only the strong survive. If you want to succeed, if you want to achieve greatness, you need to have an unbreakable mental resilience. You need to develop the iron will necessary to push through any obstacle in your path.

But let me tell you something - this isn't going to be easy. Life is going to hit you hard. It's going to throw everything it's got at you, and then some. You're going to face rejection, failure, disappointment, and heartbreak. You're going to feel like giving up, like crawling into a hole and never coming out.

But that's not the attitude of a champion. That's not the attitude of a winner. You need to have the mental toughness to push through the pain and come out the other side stronger than ever.

So how do you develop this iron will? It starts with your mindset. You need to believe in yourself and your abilities. You need to know that you have what it takes to overcome any challenge that comes your way.

But it's not just about believing in yourself. You also need to have a plan of action. You need to set goals for yourself, and then work tirelessly to achieve them. You need to be willing to put in the hard work, the late nights, the early mornings, and the sacrifice necessary to achieve greatness.

But it's not just about hard work, either. You also need to be adaptable. Life is going to throw unexpected challenges your way. You need to be able to pivot and adjust your approach to meet these challenges head-on.

And when things get tough, when you feel like giving up, remember this - you're not alone. There are other men out there who are going through the same struggles you are. Reach out to them. Lean on them for support. And know that you can get through this.

Developing an unbreakable mental resilience is not an option, it's a requirement for success. It's what separates the champions from the also-rans. So make the choice today to develop your iron will. Work on your mindset, set goals, put in the hard work, be adaptable, and lean on your support system when you need it. And when life knocks you down - and it will - get back up, dust yourself off, and keep moving forward. That's what it takes to be a true champion.

Another key element in developing unbreakable mental resilience is to embrace failure. Yes, you read that right - embrace it. Failure is not something to be feared or avoided at all costs. In fact, failure is one of the most valuable learning experiences you can have.

Every time you fail, you have the opportunity to learn something new about yourself and the situation you're in. You can use that knowledge to adjust your approach and come back stronger next time.

But here's the thing - you have to be willing to fail in the first place. You have to be willing to take risks, to put yourself out there, to try new things even if you're not sure they'll work out. If you're not willing to fail, you'll never truly reach your full potential.

So how do you embrace failure? Start by reframing your mindset. Instead of seeing failure as something to be avoided at all costs, see it as an opportunity for growth. Look at it as a chance to learn something new and improve yourself.

And when you do fail - because you will - don't beat yourself up over it. Instead, take a step back and objectively analyze what went wrong.

What can you learn from this experience? How can you use that knowledge to improve in the future?

Remember, failure is not the end. It's simply a stepping stone on the path to success. Embrace it, learn from it, and keep pushing forward.

Finally, to truly develop an iron will, you need to cultivate a strong sense of purpose. You need to have a reason for doing what you do, something that drives you and motivates you even when the going gets tough.

This sense of purpose can take many forms. It could be a desire to provide for your family, a passion for a particular cause or project, or a drive to achieve greatness in your chosen field.

Whatever it is, hold onto it. Let it be your guiding light when everything else seems dark. When you feel like giving up, remind yourself why you started in the first place. Reconnect with your sense of purpose, and use that as motivation to keep pushing forward.

And as you embark on this journey of developing unbreakable mental resilience, don't forget to take care of yourself. Mental toughness doesn't mean ignoring your emotional needs or pushing yourself to the point of burnout.

Make sure to take breaks when you need them, to engage in self-care activities that bring you joy and relaxation, and to seek out professional help if necessary. There is no shame in asking for help when you need it, and in fact, it takes a great deal of strength and courage to do so.

Remember, the road to developing an iron will is a long and arduous one, but the rewards are immeasurable. By embracing failure, cultivating a strong sense of purpose, and taking care of yourself along the way, you can achieve mental toughness beyond your wildest dreams.

And when you do, you will be able to face any challenge, overcome any obstacle, and achieve greatness in all areas of your life. So go forth, my fellow men, and develop the unbreakable mental resilience and iron will that will set you apart from the rest.

G.O.A.T Rule #3 | The Alpha Mindset: Cultivating Unstoppable Confidence and Assertiveness

> **"**
>
> *If you want to be a lion, you can't act like a lamb - cultivate an alpha mindset that exudes power, confidence, and fearlessness*

Yo, what's up? Get ready to develop the alpha mindset, because you're about to learn how to cultivate unstoppable confidence and assertiveness. If you want to make something of yourself in this world, you need to toughen up and develop an alpha mindset. Without confidence and assertiveness, you're nothing but a weakling in the eyes of others. It's time to take control and become a force to be reckoned with, starting with your mindset. So, let's dive in and learn how to cultivate an unstoppable alpha mentality.

First things first, you need to wake up to the harsh reality of the world we live in. It's a cutthroat and competitive place, and you can't expect to succeed by being passive and timid. You need to assert yourself in every situation and set clear boundaries and expectations for others. If you don't stand up for yourself, people will walk all over you like the doormat you are.

Secondly, you need to develop a winner's mentality. That means believing in yourself and your abilities, even when others doubt you. You need to have the resilience and determination to push through any obstacle that comes your way. No matter how tough things get, you can't give up. You need to keep pushing until you achieve your goals and prove all the haters wrong.

Next up, you need to take care of yourself physically and mentally. You can't be a confident and assertive alpha if you're not healthy and balanced. That means eating right, exercising regularly, and taking care of your mental health. You can't let stress and anxiety hold you back or make excuses for not taking care of yourself.

Fourthly, you need to surround yourself with other alpha-minded people. You need a tribe of like-minded individuals who will push you to be your best self. Iron sharpens iron, and you need to be around people who will challenge you and make you better. Cut the losers and negative people out of your life and only surround yourself with those who will help you grow.

Fifth, you need to be willing to take risks and make mistakes. Failure is a necessary part of the learning process. You can't be afraid of it. You need to embrace your mistakes and use them as opportunities to learn and grow. Remember, taking risks is the only way to achieve greatness.

Sixth, you need to be decisive and take action. Indecisiveness is a sign of weakness, and you can't afford to show any signs of that. You need to be able to make quick decisions and take action on them. That means having a plan and executing it with confidence.

Seventh, you need to be willing to speak your mind and stand up for what you believe in. Don't be a sheep and go along with the crowd. Be bold and unapologetic in your opinions and beliefs, even if it means being the lone voice in a sea of conformity.

Eighth, you need to be constantly learning and growing. The world is always changing, and you need to stay ahead of the curve. Read books, attend seminars, and seek out mentors who can teach you new things. Never stop learning and never become complacent.

Ninth, you need to be disciplined and focused. You can't afford to waste time on distractions and frivolous activities. You need to be laser-focused on your goals and work tirelessly towards them. You need to be willing to sacrifice and put in the hard work to achieve your dreams.

And lastly, you need to be authentic and true to yourself. Don't try to be someone you're not just to fit in or impress others. Be comfortable in your own skin and embrace your unique qualities.

This is what will set you apart from the crowd and make you truly alpha!

G.O.A.T Rule #4 | Mastering Your Body: The Importance of Physical Fitness for Dominant Men

"

Don't make excuses. Excuses are for the weak and the mediocre. You are neither.

Listen up, men. In this world, only the strong survive. And if you want to dominate in all areas of your life, you better start taking care of your body. Physical fitness isn't just a luxury, it's a necessity. And if you're not in shape, you're not going to be able to keep up with the demands of a dominant lifestyle.

Let's get real here. The world is a tough place, and it's even tougher for men. You need to be strong, both physically and mentally, if you want to make it. And the only way to get there is through hard work and discipline.

That's why physical fitness is so important. It's a reflection of your character and your ability to take control of your life. It shows that you're willing to put in the effort to become the best version of yourself. And let's face it, women want a man who takes care of himself. If you're not in shape, you're not going to be attracting the type of women you want.

But physical fitness isn't just about looking good. It's about feeling good too. Regular exercise has been proven to reduce stress, anxiety, and depression. It gives you the energy and confidence to take on the world and succeed in all areas of your life.

So what are you waiting for? Get off your ass and start working out. Follow a consistent workout routine that includes both cardiovascular exercise and weight training. And make sure you're eating a healthy diet that includes plenty of protein, vegetables, and healthy fats.

Remember, you're not just working out for your physical health. You're working out to become a dominant man who can conquer anything that comes his way. So start today, and never look back.

But let me be clear, getting in shape isn't easy. It takes hard work, dedication, and sacrifice. You're going to have to say no to that slice of pizza and that beer after work. You're going to have to wake up early and hit the gym, even when you don't feel like it. You're going to have to push yourself to your limits, and then push even harder.

But the rewards are worth it. When you're in shape, you'll feel like a king. You'll have more energy, more confidence, and more drive to succeed. You'll be able to handle anything that comes your way, and you'll do it with style and grace.

So don't make excuses. Don't say you don't have time or that you're too tired. If you want to be a dominant man, you need to take care of your body. It's the foundation of your success, and it's the only way to achieve your goals.

And let me tell you, the world needs more dominant men. Men who are strong, confident, and capable of achieving anything they set their minds to. Men who can lead, inspire, and motivate others to greatness. Men who can stand up to the challenges of life and come out victorious.

So if you want to be a dominant man, start by taking care of your body. Get in shape, eat healthy, and stay disciplined. And remember, there's no such thing as an overnight success. It takes time and effort to become the best version of yourself. But if you stay committed and keep pushing forward, you'll get there. And when you do, you'll be a force to be reckoned with.

But physical fitness is just one part of mastering your body as a dominant man. You also need to be aware of your posture, body language, and overall presence. Your body is a tool, and you need to know how to use it to your advantage.

Good posture is essential for a dominant man. It conveys confidence, strength, and authority. When you walk into a room with your head held high and your shoulders back, people take notice. It shows that you're in control of yourself and your environment.

Body language is also important. You need to be aware of your gestures, facial expressions, and tone of voice. A dominant man speaks with authority and conviction. He's not afraid to take up space or make eye contact. He commands attention with his presence and his words.

Finally, you need to be aware of your overall presence. How you dress, groom, and carry yourself all contribute to your image as a dominant man. You need to look the part if you want to play the part. Dress in clothes that fit well and flatter your body type. Keep your grooming clean and sharp. And always be aware of how you come across to others.

Mastering your body is an essential part of being a dominant man. Physical fitness, good posture, body language, and overall presence are all important aspects to consider. Remember, your body is a tool, and you need to know how to use it to your advantage. By taking care of your body and being aware of your presence, you can become a dominant force in all areas of your life. So start today and take control of your body and your destiny.

G.O.A.T Rule #5 | Money, Power, Respect: How to Command Attention

> ❝
>
> *Money, power, and respect are the keys to becoming a real man, but only if they're used to make a positive impact on the world around you.*

Alright, men, let's talk about something that every real man needs to understand: money, power, and respect. If you want to command attention and be a true alpha male in this world, you need to have these things under control. In this chapter, I'm going to teach you how to take control of your financial and social life to become a dominant force.

Let's start with money. Money is essential to living a comfortable and successful life. If you want to be a real man, you need to understand how to make money and manage it properly. You need to have a financial plan in place and stick to it. Whether you're running your own business or working for someone else, you need to be able to handle your finances like a pro.

But money isn't everything. You also need power and influence to be a real man. You need to have the ability to lead and command respect from those around you. This comes from having a strong presence and being able to communicate effectively. You need to be able to take charge and make decisions that benefit both yourself and those around you.

And speaking of respect, it's something that every real man needs to earn. You can't demand respect; you have to earn it. You need to treat others with respect and dignity, and in turn, they will respect you. This means being honest, trustworthy, and reliable. It means being a man of your word and following through on your commitments.

Now, I know that money, power, and respect can seem like daunting concepts, especially if you're just starting out in life. But the truth is, anyone can achieve these things with hard work and dedication. It's all about setting goals and working towards them every single day.

Let's dive deeper into the concept of money, power, and respect, and how they can help you become a real man in this era.

First, let's talk about money. Money is a tool that can help you achieve your goals and live the life you want. It provides financial stability, allows you to invest in yourself and your future, and gives you the freedom to make choices that align with your values. To attain financial success, you need to be willing to work hard and make smart decisions.

One way to start building wealth is to focus on increasing your income. This could mean working overtime, starting a side hustle, or taking on a new job that pays more. You also need to learn how to manage your money effectively by creating a budget, saving for emergencies, and investing in your future.

Next, let's talk about power. Power is the ability to influence others and create change. It comes from being confident in your abilities, communicating effectively, and taking control of your life. As a real man, you need to develop leadership skills that allow you to inspire and motivate others.

To gain power, you need to start by developing a strong sense of self. This means understanding your strengths and weaknesses and working on improving them. You also need to be able to communicate your vision and ideas effectively to others, and be willing to take risks to achieve your goals.

Finally, let's talk about respect. Respect is earned through your actions and the way you treat others. As a real man, you need to earn the respect of those around you by being honest, trustworthy, and reliable. You also need to be respectful towards others, even if you disagree with them.

To earn respect, you need to start by treating others the way you want to be treated. This means being kind, compassionate, and empathetic towards others. You also need to be a man of your word, and follow through on your commitments.

So, how do you bring all of these concepts together to become a real man in this era? It starts with setting goals and working towards them every day. You need to be willing to work hard and make sacrifices to achieve your dreams.

You also need to be willing to take risks and step outside of your comfort zone. This means being open to new experiences and challenges, and learning from your mistakes along the way.

Money, power, and respect are essential concepts that every real man needs to understand. By focusing on these areas, you can develop the skills and mindset needed to become a dominant force in your personal and professional life. So, start taking action today and make your dreams a reality. Remember, the journey to becoming a real man is a long and challenging one, but the rewards are well worth it.

Additionally, it's important to understand that money, power, and respect are not just about personal gain. They can also be used to help others and make a positive impact on the world around you.

As a real man, you have a responsibility to use your influence and resources for good. This could mean volunteering your time and money to charitable causes, mentoring others, or using your platform to bring attention to important issues.

Furthermore, it's crucial to understand that the pursuit of money, power, and respect should never come at the expense of your values or morals. It's easy to get caught up in the idea of success and lose sight of what's truly important.

Always strive to be true to yourself and stay grounded in your beliefs. This will not only help you earn the respect of others, but also allow you to live a fulfilling and meaningful life.

Lastly, it's important to remember that the journey to becoming a real man is not a linear one. There will be setbacks, failures, and obstacles along the way. It's how you handle these challenges that will define your character and determine your success.

So, if you want to be a real man in this era, you need to take control of your financial and social life. You need to understand the importance of money, power, and respect and work towards achieving them every single day. Don't let anyone hold you back, and don't be afraid to take risks. Remember, the greatest rewards in life often come from taking the biggest risks.

G.O.A.T Rule #6 | Quit Being a Softie: Unleashing Your Inner Savage and Becoming a Force to be Reckoned with.

> **"**
>
> *Becoming a savage means tapping into the primal instincts that make us human - it's about unleashing the beast within*

Alright, let's cut the bullshit and get real. If you're looking for a way to tap into your animal instincts and become a true savage, then you've come to the right place. I'm here to help you unleash your inner beast.

Let me tell you something straight up, being a real man in this era is no easy feat. Society has been feminized and emasculated, and too many men have lost touch with their primal instincts. But I'm not here to make excuses or pity you. I'm here to motivate you and show you how to become the alpha male that you were meant to be.

First off, let's talk about animal instincts. We all have them, but most people suppress them or don't even realize they exist. Your animal instincts are what drive you to fight, hunt, and protect. They are what give you that killer instinct that separates the winners from the losers.

To tap into your animal instincts, you need to embrace your primal nature. Stop being a soft, sensitive wimp and start being a savage. That means lifting weights, training martial arts, and taking risks. You need to be physically and mentally strong, and you need to be willing to do whatever it takes to succeed.

To be a true savage, you need to have a deep understanding of yourself and the world around you. You need to be self-aware and recognize your strengths and weaknesses. You need to embrace your physical and mental abilities and constantly work on improving them. You also need to understand that the world is not a fair place, and that sometimes you need to take risks and make sacrifices to get what you want.

But being a savage isn't just about physical strength. It's also about mental toughness. You need to be able to handle the harsh realities of this world and not let them break you. That means embracing pain and discomfort, and not shying away from difficult situations. It means being resilient in the face of failure and rejection, and always pushing forward no matter what.

Now, I know that some people might say that this kind of mentality is toxic or harmful. But let me tell you something, the real world is not a safe space. It's a jungle, and only the strong survive. If you want to be a real man and succeed in this world, you need to be willing to fight for what you want and take what is rightfully yours.

If you're reading this book, then you're probably looking for a way to become a real man. And let me tell you something, being a real man isn't about being politically correct or following society's rules. It's about being a savage and doing whatever it takes to win. Let's dive deep into what it means to be a savage in today's world. It's important to acknowledge that the definition of a real man or a savage varies from person to person.

Now, it's important to note that being a savage doesn't mean being a jerk or intentionally hurting others. It's about being confident and assertive, but also having empathy and respect for others. You should strive to be a leader and inspire others, rather than tearing them down. Being a savage means standing up for what you believe in and being true to yourself, but also recognizing that others have their own beliefs and values.

Another important aspect of being a savage is having a purpose. You need to have a clear vision of what you want to achieve in life and work towards it every day. This doesn't mean that you need to have everything figured out, but you should have a general direction and be actively working towards it. Having a purpose gives you a sense of direction and meaning, and it helps you stay focused and motivated.

Now that we've established what it means to be a true savage, let's talk about how to tap into your animal instincts and become one. The first step is to recognize that you have these instincts, and to embrace them fully. This means letting go of societal norms and expectations, and trusting your gut instincts instead.

One way to tap into your animal instincts is through physical training. This could be weightlifting, martial arts, or any other activity that challenges you physically. Not only will this make you stronger and more physically capable, but it will also boost your confidence and give you a sense of control over your body.

Another way to tap into your animal instincts is through mental training. This could be meditation, visualization, or any other activity that helps you develop mental toughness and resilience. By strengthening your mind, you'll be better equipped to handle difficult situations and overcome obstacles.

But perhaps the most important way to tap into your animal instincts is through experience. You need to put yourself in situations that challenge you and push you outside of your comfort zone. This could be traveling to a new country, trying a new hobby, or taking on a new job. By exposing yourself to new experiences, you'll learn more about yourself and develop the skills and confidence needed to thrive in this world.

It's also important to recognize that being a true savage is not just about you. It's about being a positive force in the world and helping others. This means having empathy and compassion for others, and using your skills and abilities to make a difference in the world.

G.O.A.T Rule #7 | Stop Being a Weakling: Obliterating Your Insecurities by Dominating Self-Doubt and Fear

> *Pain is temporary, but regret lasts forever. Real men are willing to endure the pain of growth to avoid the regret of stagnation.*

Listen up, warrior. If you want to be a real man in this world, you need to stop being a little wuss and start crushing your weaknesses. And let me tell you, self-doubt and fear are two of the biggest weaknesses that men face. These emotions will eat away at your confidence and make you look weak in front of others. And nobody wants to be seen as weak, right?

Self-doubt is a disease that spreads like wildfire. It will hold you back and prevent you from achieving your goals. And fear? Fear is just a lame excuse to avoid taking action and facing your problems head-on. But here's the thing, real men don't make excuses. They take action and overcome their weaknesses.

So, if you want to be a real man, you need to stop being a little baby and learn how to push through your fears and take action, even when you're scared. And you need to develop the confidence to trust your instincts and make decisions without second-guessing yourself. Stop being a little boy and start being a man who takes control of his life.

Now, I know it's tough to overcome self-doubt and fear, but the first step is to recognize that they're holding you back. You need to acknowledge that you're weak and start working on overcoming those weaknesses. And let me tell you, there's no room for being a coward in this world.

One technique that I use to overcome self-doubt is to focus on my strengths. Instead of dwelling on my weaknesses and what I can't do, I focus on what I'm good at and what I can do. This helps me build confidence and reminds me that I'm capable of achieving my goals.

Another technique is to take action, even when I'm scared. The more I take action and push through my fears, the less scared I become. And the more confident I become in my ability to handle challenges and overcome obstacles.

So, if you want to be a real man in this world, start by crushing your weaknesses. Overcome your self-doubt and fear, focus on your strengths, and take action, even when you're scared. And don't be a little baby about it. It won't be easy, but nothing worth having ever is. Remember, real men don't make excuses. They take action and overcome their weaknesses. So, what kind of man do you want to be?

But let's not forget, being a real man also means knowing when to be assertive and take charge. Real men don't let others walk all over them. They stand up for themselves and those they care about. So, don't be afraid to be assertive and take control when necessary.

Alright, let me break it down for you even further. The truth is, self-doubt and fear are ingrained in our biology. They're natural survival mechanisms that helped our ancestors avoid danger and stay alive. But in today's world, these same mechanisms can hold us back and prevent us from achieving our goals.

That's why it's so important to recognize that self-doubt and fear are just thoughts and emotions. They're not real. They're just your brain's way of trying to protect you from perceived threats. But the thing is, most of the time those threats are imaginary. They're not actually happening in the present moment.

So, the first step in overcoming self-doubt and fear is to recognize that they're just thoughts and emotions. They're not reality. Once you can do that, you can start to question those thoughts and challenge them.

For example, let's say you're about to give a presentation at work, and you're feeling really nervous. Your brain might be telling you things like "I'm going to mess up" or "Everyone is going to laugh at me". But the reality is, those things probably aren't going to happen. Most likely, your presentation will go just fine, and no one will even remember it in a few days.

So, when you start to feel those thoughts and emotions, take a step back and ask yourself, "Is this really true? Am I really in danger?" Chances are, the answer is no.

Another thing you can do to overcome self-doubt and fear is to practice self-compassion. Realize that everyone experiences these feelings at some point. You're not alone. And it's okay to feel scared or unsure. Give yourself permission to be imperfect and make mistakes. And remember, failure is not the end of the world. It's just a learning experience.

Now, let's talk about fear. Fear is a powerful emotion, but it's also a choice. You can choose to let your fears control you, or you can choose to face them head-on. And the more you face your fears, the less power they will have over you.

One technique that I use to overcome fear is called exposure therapy. Basically, you expose yourself to the thing you're afraid of in a safe and controlled environment. For example, if you're afraid of public speaking, you might start by giving a speech in front of a small group of friends or family. Then, gradually work your way up to larger groups and more challenging situations.

Another technique is to reframe your fears as opportunities. Instead of seeing them as something to avoid, see them as a chance to grow and learn. Embrace the challenge and push yourself out of your comfort zone.

So, to sum it up, if you want to be a real man in this world, you need to learn how to overcome self-doubt and fear. Recognize that they're just thoughts and emotions, challenge them, practice self-compassion, and face your fears head-on. It won't be easy, but it will be worth it.

And remember, being a real man is not about being fearless. It's about having the courage to face your fears and take action in spite of them. So, what are you waiting for? Start crushing your weaknesses and becoming the man you were meant to be.

One thing to keep in mind is that overcoming self-doubt and fear is not a one-time event. It's a lifelong process. Even the most confident and successful people have moments of self-doubt and fear. But the difference is, they don't let those feelings hold them back. They recognize them for what they are and push through them.

Another important aspect of overcoming self-doubt and fear is to surround yourself with positive and supportive people. Real men don't tear each other down. They lift each other up. Find friends, mentors, and role models who will encourage you and push you to be your best self. And don't be afraid to ask for help when you need it.

It's also important to take care of your physical health. Exercise, eat well, and get enough sleep. When your body is healthy, your mind is healthy too. And a healthy mind is better equipped to handle challenges and overcome self-doubt and fear.

Finally, remember that being a real man is not about conforming to someone else's idea of masculinity. It's about being true to yourself and living a life that is authentic and fulfilling. Don't compare yourself to others or try to live up to unrealistic expectations. Define your own values and goals, and work towards them with determination and purpose.

Crushing your weaknesses and overcoming self-doubt and fear is essential if you want to be a real man in this world. It takes courage, perseverance, and a willingness to push yourself out of your comfort zone. But the rewards are well worth it. You'll gain confidence, self-respect, and the ability to live a life that is authentic and fulfilling. So, what are you waiting for?

Start taking action today and become the man you were meant to be.

G.O.A.T Rule #8 | The Art of Not Being a P*ssy: Mastering Your Emotions and Living Life on Your Terms

"

Emotions are a double-edged sword. Learn to wield them with precision, and you'll be unstoppable.

Listen up, emotions ain't a weakness, they can be your strength if you know how to use them. But don't be a slave to your emotions, you gotta control them. And being a real man ain't about being a macho tough guy, it's about being confident, respectful, and a leader. Take care of yourself physically, mentally, and emotionally, set goals, and take risks. And don't forget about emotional intelligence, mental fortitude, and spiritual depth. You gotta cultivate these qualities, challenge yourself, and find purpose beyond just material success. So go out there and unleash your inner beast, but always stay true to yourself, man.

First and foremost, let's address the elephant in the room: emotions. A real man isn't afraid to feel them, but he also knows how to control them. Don't let society fool you into thinking that being emotional is a weakness. In fact, it's the complete opposite. Emotions can be a source of great strength and motivation if you know how to use them to your advantage.

However, there's a fine line between being emotional and being a slave to your emotions. You must master your emotions, not the other way around. This means being in control of your actions and reactions, even when your emotions are running high. It means channeling your anger, frustration, and sadness into something productive, rather than letting them consume you.

Now, let's talk about what it means to be a real man in today's world. It's not about being a macho tough guy who walks around with his chest puffed out, looking for a fight. It's about being confident in who you are and what you stand for. It's about being respectful to others, but not letting anyone walk all over you. It's about being a leader, not a follower.

But being a real man isn't just about how you act towards others. It's also about how you treat yourself. Are you taking care of your physical health? Are you constantly striving to improve yourself mentally and emotionally? Are you setting goals and working towards them every day? These are the things that separate the real men from the boys.

But here's the thing, being a real man doesn't mean you have to be a pushover or a doormat. You gotta stand up for yourself and what you believe in, even if it means going against the crowd. And yeah, sometimes that means being politically incorrect or using colorful language. But that's just part of being a real man, speaking your mind and not giving a damn about what anyone else thinks.

And let's not forget about the ladies. Being a real man means treating women with respect and dignity, but also being confident and assertive in your approach. It's about being a gentleman, but not a pushover. So go ahead, unleash your inner beast and become the man you were meant to be. Just remember, it's not for the faint of heart.

So, how do you unleash your inner beast and master your emotions? It starts with being honest with yourself. Are you living up to your full potential? Are you using your emotions to fuel your drive, or are they holding you back? Once you've answered these questions, it's time to take action.

Start by setting goals for yourself, both short-term and long-term. Write them down and create a plan of action to achieve them. Don't be afraid to take risks and step outside of your comfort zone. Embrace your emotions, but don't let them control you. Use them to fuel your drive and motivation.

Being a real man in today's world isn't about being a tough guy or a macho man. It's about being confident, respectful, and a leader. It's about taking care of yourself and constantly striving to improve. Unleashing your inner beast and mastering your emotions starts with being honest with yourself and taking action.

Now, let's dive deeper into what it really means to be a real man in today's world.

One of the biggest misconceptions about being a real man is that it's all about physical strength and dominance. While physical strength is certainly an important aspect of masculinity, it's not the only one. True masculinity also involves emotional intelligence, mental fortitude, and spiritual depth.

Emotional intelligence is the ability to recognize, understand, and manage your own emotions, as well as the emotions of others. A real man doesn't shy away from his emotions, but he doesn't let them control him either. He's able to channel his emotions into something productive and positive, rather than letting them consume him.

Mental fortitude is the ability to push through obstacles and challenges, even when the going gets tough. A real man doesn't give up when things get difficult. Instead, he uses his inner strength and resilience to overcome adversity and come out stronger on the other side.

Spiritual depth involves a sense of purpose and meaning beyond just the physical realm. A real man has a strong sense of values and beliefs that guide his actions and decisions. He has a deep connection to something greater than himself, whether it's his faith, his family, or his community.

So, how do you cultivate these qualities and become a real man in today's world? It starts with taking care of yourself, both physically and mentally. Make sure you're getting enough sleep, exercise, and healthy food. Take time to practice mindfulness, meditation, or other forms of self-care that help you stay grounded and centered.

Next, focus on developing your emotional intelligence. This means being aware of your own emotions and how they affect you, as well as being able to empathize with others and understand their perspectives. It also means being able to manage your emotions in a healthy way, rather than letting them control you.

To build mental fortitude, challenge yourself to step outside of your comfort zone on a regular basis. Set ambitious goals for yourself and work towards them consistently, even when it feels difficult or impossible. Surround yourself with supportive people who believe in you and encourage you to be your best self.

Finally, cultivate spiritual depth by finding meaning and purpose in your life. This might involve exploring your faith or spirituality, volunteering in your community, or pursuing a passion that brings you joy and fulfillment. Whatever it is, make sure it aligns with your values and beliefs and gives you a sense of purpose beyond just material success.

Being a real man in today's world is about much more than just physical strength or toughness. It involves emotional intelligence, mental fortitude, and spiritual depth. By taking care of yourself, developing these qualities, and aligning your actions with your values and beliefs, you can unleash your inner beast and become the best version of yourself. So go out there and be a real man, but remember to stay true to yourself and always be authentic.

G.O.A.T Rule #9 | Get Your Sh*t Together: Uncovering Your Purpose and Igniting Your Passion on the Path to Unstoppable Greatness.

> **"**
>
> *Stop wasting your life on meaningless distractions and start uncovering your purpose and fueling your passion to become truly unstoppable*

Alright, listen up. It's time to get your sh*t together and uncover your purpose. You want to be a real man in this world? Then you need to ignite your passion and pursue greatness. It's not going to be easy, but nothing worth having ever is.

Let me tell you something, being a real man in this era is harder than it's ever been before. You're bombarded with distractions, propaganda, and social pressure to be someone you're not. But you know what? None of that matters. The only thing that matters is your drive and your determination to be the best version of yourself.

First things first, you need to uncover your purpose. What drives you? What motivates you? What makes you tick? If you can answer these questions, then you're on the right track. Your purpose will give you direction, it will give you focus, and it will give you something to strive towards. Without purpose, you're just wandering aimlessly, and that's no way to live.

But here's the harsh reality - finding your purpose isn't easy. It takes time, effort, and a lot of self-reflection. You need to be honest with yourself and acknowledge your strengths and weaknesses. You need to be willing to take risks and step out of your comfort zone. You need to be open to new experiences and opportunities. It's not going to happen overnight, but it will happen if you stay committed to the journey.

Now, let's talk about passion. You can have all the purpose in the world, but if you're not passionate about it, then it's pointless. Passion is what fuels your purpose. It's what gets you out of bed in the morning and keeps you up late at night. It's what makes you feel alive.

But here's the thing - passion doesn't just fall into your lap. You need to actively seek it out. You need to try new things, explore new interests, and find what resonates with you. It might take some trial and error, but that's okay. It's all part of the journey.

And finally, let's talk about greatness. What does it mean to be great? It means being the best version of yourself. It means pushing yourself to your limits and beyond. It means never settling for mediocrity.

But here's the truth - greatness isn't for everyone. It takes hard work, discipline, and sacrifice. You need to be willing to put in the effort and make the necessary changes to your lifestyle. You need to be willing to prioritize your goals over short-term pleasure. It's not easy, but it's worth it.

And let's be clear - being a real man doesn't mean conforming to some outdated stereotype. It's not about being macho or dominant. It's about being confident in who you are and what you stand for. It's about being resilient in the face of adversity. It's about being a leader, not a follower.

But being a leader doesn't mean being perfect. It means being willing to make mistakes and learn from them. It means taking responsibility for your actions and owning up to your failures. It means being vulnerable and authentic.

And that's the thing - being a real man means being authentic. It means being true to yourself and your values. It means not pretending to be someone you're not just to fit in. It means having the courage to stand up for what you believe in, even if it's unpopular.

So, how do you become a real man in this era? It starts with getting your sh*t together. It starts with uncovering your purpose and igniting your passion. It starts with pursuing greatness and being authentic.

But it also starts with recognizing that you're not alone. There are other men out there who are on the same journey as you. Seek out mentors, friends, and community who share your values and can support you along the way.

And remember, this journey is not a destination. It's a lifelong pursuit. You will face setbacks, obstacles, and challenges along the way. But if you stay committed to the process, you will emerge stronger and more resilient than ever before.

So, to all the men out there who are ready to step up and be real men in this world - I challenge you to get your sh*t together. Uncover your purpose. Ignite your passion. Pursue greatness. And above all, be authentic. The world needs more real men like you.

So, what's the bottom line? If you want to be a real man in this world, then you need to get your sh*t together. You need to uncover your purpose, ignite your passion, and pursue greatness. It's not going to be easy, but it will be worth it. The world needs more real men - are you up for the challenge?

G.O.A.T Rule #10 | Life is Tough, So Get Tougher: The Blueprint to Conquering Adversity

> **"**
>
> *Adversity is a test of character - toughen up and show the world what you're made of!*

Alright, listen up. Life is tough, but that's no excuse to be weak. If you want to be a real man in this world, you need to toughen up and conquer adversity. It's not going to be easy, but nothing worth having ever is.

Let's get real for a minute. Life is not fair. It will knock you down, beat you up, and leave you for dead. But you know what? That's just the way it is. You can either sit there and cry about it, or you can toughen up and fight back.

And that's the thing - being a real man means being a fighter. It means having the strength and resilience to take on whatever life throws at you. It means not giving up when the going gets tough. It means standing up for what you believe in, even when it's unpopular.

But here's the harsh reality - being a fighter is not easy. It takes guts, determination, and a whole lot of grit. It means putting in the work, day in and day out, to build the kind of strength that can withstand any challenge.

So, how do you toughen up and conquer adversity? It starts with mindset. You need to shift your perspective from victim to victor. You need to stop making excuses and start taking responsibility for your life. You need to stop playing it safe and start taking risks.

But mindset is just the beginning. You also need to take action. You need to push yourself outside of your comfort zone, and challenge yourself to do things you never thought possible. You need to embrace the struggle, and use it as fuel to become stronger.

And let's be clear - toughness doesn't mean being a brute. It means having emotional intelligence, being vulnerable, and seeking help when you need it. It means being a leader, not a bully. It means being confident in who you are and what you stand for.

So, to all the men out there who want to be real men in this world - I challenge you to toughen up and conquer adversity. It won't be easy, but it will be worth it. Remember, life is tough, but so are you.

To truly conquer adversity, you need to understand that failure is not just a part of the process - it's an opportunity to toughen up and come back stronger. Real men don't just get up once or twice, they get up every time they fall down. Failure is not a defeat, it's a lesson, so stop whining and start learning!

But to be a real man who conquers adversity, you need to be willing to face your fears head-on. Fear is what separates the men from the boys. If you're too scared to fail, then you'll never have the guts to succeed. So, man up and take some risks!

And let's be brutally honest - life is not just about finding meaning and purpose. It's about surviving and thriving in a world that doesn't care about your feelings. Real men don't just toughen up to pursue their passions and goals, they do it to survive and thrive in a world that's constantly trying to beat them down.

So, stop wasting time trying to find your purpose and start toughening up for the real world. Take some time to figure out what you're truly made of, and push yourself beyond your limits.

But the most important thing to remember is that you are not entitled to anything in this world. You need to earn your place, your respect, and your success. Don't just seek out mentors and community to support you, seek out competition to push you to be better.

In the end, being a real man who conquers adversity is not about being perfect. It's about being resilient, courageous, and authentic.

It's about being willing to take risks, embrace the struggle, and dominate your competition.

So, to all the men out there who want to be real men in this world - I challenge you to get tough and conquer adversity. It won't be easy, but it will be worth it. And remember, you are not entitled to anything - you need to earn it. So, get out there and earn your greatness!

G.O.A.T Rule #11 | Master the Battle Within: How to Develop a Warrior's Mindset and Achieve Victory in All Areas of Life

> **"**
>
> *To be a true warrior, you must first conquer your own mind. Mental toughness is the weapon that will help you achieve victory in all areas of life*

Alright, gentlemen, let's talk about developing a warrior's mindset. It's easy to get complacent and accept the status quo, but if you want to achieve victory in all areas of life, you need to step up and develop a mindset of mental toughness, resilience, and grit.

So, how do you do that? It's not going to be easy, but it is going to be worth it. Here are some key steps you can take to develop a warrior's mindset and become unstoppable in all areas of life.

First and foremost, you need to embrace the struggle. Life is not supposed to be easy, and it's not supposed to be comfortable. Real men don't shy away from challenges - they embrace them. Every obstacle you face is an opportunity to toughen up and become stronger. Embrace the struggle and push through the pain.

Secondly, you need to take ownership of your life. Real men don't make excuses or blame others for their problems. They take responsibility for their situation and work hard to overcome any obstacle in their path. You need to recognize that you are in control of your life and that you have the power to change it for the better.

Thirdly, you need to develop mental toughness. This means being able to push through the pain, face your fears, and never give up. Mental toughness is not something you're born with - it's something you develop through hard work and dedication. One of the best ways to develop mental toughness is to practice visualization exercises. Picture yourself overcoming obstacles and achieving your goals, and repeat positive affirmations to yourself every day.

Fourthly, you need to set clear goals for yourself. Real men don't just drift through life aimlessly. They have a clear vision of what they want to achieve, and they work hard every day to make it happen. Setting goals helps you stay focused and motivated, and gives you a clear direction to work towards.

Fifthly, you need to surround yourself with other warriors. Real men don't just toughen up on their own - they have a community of like-minded individuals who support and encourage them. Seek out mentors, friends, and community who share your values and can support you along the way.

Sixthly, you need to learn from failure. Real men don't give up after failing once or twice. They use failure as a learning opportunity and come back even stronger. Failure is not the end - it's just a temporary setback on the road to success. Embrace failure and use it as a stepping stone to success.

Seventhly, you need to have a strong work ethic. Real men don't expect success to be handed to them on a silver platter. They work hard every day to achieve their goals and never stop pushing themselves to be better. Develop a strong work ethic by setting high standards for yourself and never settling for anything less.

Eighthly, you need to be willing to take risks. Real men don't play it safe - they take calculated risks and embrace the unknown. Taking risks is a key part of achieving success, and you need to be willing to step out of your comfort zone in order to achieve your goals.

Ninthly, you need to be adaptable. Life is unpredictable, and things don't always go according to plan. Real men are able to adapt to new situations and come out on top. Develop adaptability by being open-minded and flexible, and by staying calm and focused in the face of uncertainty.

Tenthly, you need to never settle. Real men don't just achieve their goals and then stop. They set new goals and continue pushing themselves to be better every day. Never settle for mediocrity - always strive for greatness.

Developing a warrior's mindset is all about embracing the struggle, taking ownership of your life, developing mental toughness, setting clear goals, surrounding yourself with other warriors, learning from failure, having a strong work ethic, being willing to take risks, being adaptable, and never settling for mediocrity.

It's not going to be easy, but if you're willing to put in the work, you can develop a warrior's mindset and achieve victory in all areas of life. Remember, it's not about being perfect - it's about being resilient, courageous, and authentic. It's about being willing to take risks, embrace the struggle, and pursue your passions.

So, to all the men out there who want to be warriors in this world - I challenge you to take action and develop a warrior's mindset. It won't be easy, but it will be worth it. And remember, you are not alone. We are all in this together. So let's rise up, face our fears, and conquer our inner battles.

G.O.A.T Rule #12 | The Dominant Mindset: Unleashing Your Unstoppable Force, Building Your Confidence, and Dominating Your Industry and Life with Utter Domination

> "
>
> *Like a lion hunting its prey, unleash your unstoppable force and dominate your industry with unmatched power and authority.*

Alright, let's dive deeper into what it truly means to have a dominant mindset and how you can achieve it. But first, let me be clear - this is not for the weak-hearted or the timid. If you want to dominate your industry and life, you must be willing to put in the work and make the sacrifices necessary to achieve your goals.

To develop a dominant mindset, you must first identify your core values and beliefs. What do you stand for? What are your non-negotiables? Once you have a clear understanding of your values, you must live and breathe them in all aspects of your life. Your values are your guiding principles that will help you stay focused and grounded on your journey towards dominance.

But values alone are not enough. You must also have a clear and compelling vision of what you want to achieve. A vision that excites and motivates you, and that you are willing to put in the work to make it a reality. Your vision should be specific and measurable, with clear goals and action steps to achieve them.

Another important aspect of developing a dominant mindset is to surround yourself with people who share your values and drive. Seek out mentors, coaches, and peers who have achieved the level of success you aspire to, and learn from their experiences. A strong support network will keep you motivated and accountable to your goals, and will provide a sounding board for new ideas and strategies.

But perhaps the most critical element of a dominant mindset is mental toughness. You must be willing to face your fears, embrace the struggle, and never give up on your goals. Failure is not an option for those who seek dominance - it is simply a learning opportunity to adjust and adapt your strategies.

To develop mental toughness, you must train your mind just as you would train your body. Challenge yourself with difficult tasks and push yourself out of your comfort zone. Develop a positive mindset and use positive self-talk to overcome negative thoughts and doubts.

In addition, physical fitness is also an essential component of a dominant mindset. Your body and mind are connected, and a strong body will help you maintain mental focus and clarity. Incorporate regular exercise into your routine, eat a healthy diet, and prioritize sleep and recovery.

But let's be clear - dominance is not about being ruthless or stepping on others to get ahead. It is about having a clear vision, strong values, mental toughness, and a willingness to work hard to achieve your goals. You must be willing to lift others up and contribute to your community while still maintaining your drive for success.

Developing a dominant mindset requires a deep understanding of your values, a clear and compelling vision, a strong support network, mental toughness, physical fitness, and a drive to succeed. It won't be easy, and it won't happen overnight. But if you're willing to put in the work and make the sacrifices necessary, you can achieve greatness in all areas of your life. Dominate your industry and your life with a dominant mindset that can't be stopped.

But let's be real - even with all the right tools and strategies, there will be setbacks and obstacles on your journey towards dominance. That's why it's important to have a mindset of resilience and adaptability.

When things don't go as planned, don't give up or get discouraged. Instead, use the situation as an opportunity to learn, grow, and pivot your strategies if necessary. Failure is only final if you give up, so keep pushing forward and never let setbacks derail your progress.

And when you do achieve success, don't become complacent or rest on your laurels. Continue to push yourself to new heights and set even bigger goals. Dominance is not a destination - it's a journey that requires constant growth and improvement.

In addition, to truly dominate your industry and your life, you must also have a strong sense of self-awareness. Understand your strengths and weaknesses, and be willing to ask for help when needed. Identify your blind spots and seek out feedback from others to continually improve.

But self-awareness also means understanding your own biases and limitations. Don't let your ego or pride blind you to new opportunities or perspectives. Stay open-minded and willing to learn from others, even if they don't share your values or beliefs.

Finally, remember that dominance is not just about personal success - it's also about making a positive impact on the world around you. Use your success and influence to give back to your community and contribute to causes that align with your values. In doing so, you will not only achieve greatness in your own life, but also leave a lasting legacy of positive change.

So, to all the aspiring dominators out there - develop a mindset of resilience, self-awareness, and contribution. Use your values, vision, and mental toughness to dominate your industry and your life with unstoppable force. And remember, success is not final and failure is not fatal - what matters most is the journey you take towards dominance.

G.O.A.T Rule #13 | Hustle and Grind: How to Finally Get Sh*t Done and Stop Being a Loser

If you want to be a winner, you have to be willing to do what losers aren't. That means putting in the work and grinding every day.

Alright, let's dive even deeper into this topic. If you want to be a real man in this world, then you need to understand that the only way to achieve greatness is through hustle and grind. There's no shortcut, no magic formula, no easy way out. You need to put in the work, day in and day out, until you reach your goals. And that means working harder than anyone else.

The harsh reality is that the world doesn't owe you anything. You're not entitled to success, respect, or admiration. You need to earn it through hard work and determination. If you want to be a real man, you need to be willing to suffer, endure pain, and push yourself to the limit and beyond. You need to be relentless in your pursuit of greatness, and never settle for mediocrity.

Now, let's talk about the specific steps you need to take to hustle and grind your way to success. The first step is to define your goals. This means being crystal clear on what you want to achieve in life, and what your long-term aspirations are. Once you have a clear picture of where you want to go, you can start creating a plan to get there.

The second step is to develop a strong work ethic. This means being willing to put in the time, effort, and energy required to achieve your goals. It means being disciplined and focused, and never giving up in the face of obstacles or setbacks. It also means being willing to learn from failure and use it as a stepping stone to success.

The third step is to surround yourself with greatness. This means finding mentors, coaches, and other successful individuals who can help guide you on your journey. It also means building a network of like-minded individuals who share your values and aspirations. You need to be constantly learning from others, taking in their wisdom and advice, and using it to fuel your hustle and grind.

The fourth step is to stay motivated. This means finding your inner drive and using it to fuel your hustle and grind. It means surrounding yourself with positive influences and staying committed to your goals no matter what. It also means celebrating your successes and using them as motivation to push even harder.

But here's the thing: hustle and grind is not just about working hard. It's also about working smart. You need to be strategic, disciplined, and focused in your approach. You need to be willing to make sacrifices, say no to distractions, and put in the extra effort required to achieve your goals. You need to be constantly refining your approach, testing new strategies, and adjusting your plan as you go.

And let's be real: there will be times when it sucks. There will be times when you feel exhausted, overwhelmed, and discouraged. But that's when you need to dig deep and find the strength to keep going. That's when you need to remind yourself why you're doing this, and why it's worth it. That's when you need to draw on your inner reserves of resilience, determination, and grit.

If you want to be a real man in this world, you need to embrace the hustle and grind. You need to be willing to put in the work, day in and day out, until you reach your goals. You need to define your goals, develop a strong work ethic, surround yourself with greatness, and stay motivated. You need to be strategic, disciplined, and focused in your approach. And most importantly, you need to be relentless in your pursuit of greatness. So go out there and hustle your way to success, and show the world what a real man looks like.

But let's be even more brutally honest here. The truth is that most people will never achieve greatness. Most people will never be real men. Most people will settle for mediocrity, complacency, and comfort. And that's fine, if that's what they want. But if you're reading this, then I know that's not what you want.

You want more. You want to be more. You want to achieve greatness and leave a lasting legacy. And the only way to do that is through hustle and grind. You need to be willing to put in the work, even when it hurts. You need to be willing to sacrifice short-term pleasures for long-term gains. You need to be willing to endure pain, discomfort, and setbacks.

The reality is that there are no shortcuts to success. There are no hacks, no magic formulas, no easy way out. If you want to be a real man, you need to earn it through hard work and determination. You need to be willing to suffer for your dreams, and never give up no matter what.

But here's the thing: the rewards are worth it. When you achieve greatness, when you reach your goals, when you become a real man, you will experience a sense of fulfillment and satisfaction that most people will never know. You will leave a lasting legacy that will inspire others to follow in your footsteps. You will be remembered as someone who didn't settle for mediocrity, who didn't give up when it got tough, who didn't compromise on his values and principles.

So don't be one of the crowd. Don't be one of the sheep who settle for less than they're capable of. Be a real man. Embrace the hustle and grind. Define your goals, develop a strong work ethic, surround yourself with greatness, and stay motivated. Be strategic, disciplined, and focused in your approach. And most importantly, be relentless in your pursuit of greatness.

G.O.A.T Rule #14 | Escape the Matrix: Breaking Free from the Illusion of Mediocrity and Living Your Best Life

> "
>
> *The matrix is real, and it's all around us. But the only way to break free is to wake up and realize that you're in it*

Alright, let's get real here. The world we live in is not what it seems. We've been fed lies and illusions our entire lives. From the media to the education system, everything is designed to keep us trapped in the matrix of mediocrity. But if you want to be a real man and live your best life, then you need to wake up and escape the matrix.

The first step is to realize that the world is not what it seems. The media tells us what to think, what to wear, what to eat, and how to live. But all of it is designed to keep us trapped in a cycle of mediocrity. We're told to go to school, get a job, get married, have kids, retire, and die. But that's not living, that's just existing.

Real men reject the illusions of mediocrity and carve out their own path in life. They don't follow the herd, they lead it. They don't settle for less than they're capable of, they strive for greatness. They don't live in the matrix, they break free from it.

The second step is to reject the illusions of mediocrity. You need to realize that the life you've been sold is a lie. You don't have to go to college, get a job, and work for someone else for 40 years. You can be an entrepreneur, start your own business, and create your own wealth. You can travel the world, meet new people, and have new experiences. You can be whoever you want to be, do whatever you want to do, and live however you want to live.

But to do that, you need to break free from the illusions that have been fed to you your entire life. You need to reject the status quo and embrace your own vision for your life. You need to be willing to take risks, make sacrifices, and work hard to achieve your dreams.

The third step is to embrace the harsh reality of what it takes to escape the matrix. You need to be willing to suffer, to sacrifice, and to struggle. Real men don't have it easy, they earn it. They don't make excuses, they make results. They don't complain, they conquer.

The truth is, breaking free from the matrix is not easy. It's a long and difficult journey that will test your strength, your courage, and your willpower. But it's worth it. When you break free, you will experience a sense of liberation and empowerment that few people ever know. You will be free to pursue your dreams, follow your passions, and live life on your own terms.

So if you want to be a real man and live your best life, then wake up and escape the matrix. Reject the illusions of mediocrity, embrace your own vision for your life, and be willing to suffer, sacrifice, and struggle to achieve your dreams. The world is waiting for you to break free and become the man you were meant to be.

Let me be clear: breaking free from the matrix is not for the faint of heart. It's not for those who are content with a mediocre life. It's for those who are willing to take risks, make sacrifices, and fight for their dreams.

Real men don't settle for less than they're capable of. They don't let fear, doubt, or insecurity hold them back. They don't let the opinions of others dictate their path in life. They follow their own path, regardless of the obstacles that stand in their way.

The truth is, the matrix is designed to keep us trapped in a cycle of mediocrity. It's designed to make us conform, to keep us in line, and to prevent us from achieving our full potential. But the real tragedy is that most people don't even realize they're in the matrix. They go through life on autopilot, never questioning the status quo, never challenging their beliefs, and never pursuing their dreams.

Real men are different. They see the world for what it is, not what they're told it is. They question everything, challenge everything, and never settle for less than they're capable of. They don't just exist, they live. They don't just survive, they thrive.

If you want to be a real man and live your best life, then you need to break free from the matrix. You need to wake up and realize that everything you've been taught is a lie. You need to reject the illusions of mediocrity and embrace your own vision for your life. You need to be willing to take risks, make sacrifices, and fight for your dreams.

It won't be easy. You'll face obstacles, setbacks, and challenges along the way. You'll have to deal with fear, doubt, and insecurity. You'll have to step out of your comfort zone and face your fears head-on. But if you're willing to do the work, if you're willing to fight for your dreams, then the rewards will be worth it.

When you break free from the matrix, you'll experience a sense of liberation and empowerment that few people ever know. You'll be free to pursue your passions, follow your dreams, and live life on your own terms. You'll be the master of your own destiny, the captain of your own ship, and the architect of your own future.

So wake up, break free, and live your best life. The world is waiting for you to become the man you were meant to be.

G.O.A.T Rule #15 | Man Up: Own Your Life and Stop Making Excuses

> **"**
>
> *Excuses are like quicksand - the more you make them, the deeper you sink. Real men don't let themselves get stuck in the mud of mediocrity*

The truth is, making excuses is a cowardly act. It's the easy way out. It's a way to avoid taking responsibility for your life and your actions. And it's a surefire way to live a mediocre life.

Real men don't make excuses. They take ownership of their lives and their actions. They don't wait for someone else to give them permission or motivation - they create their own opportunities for success.

And if you're not willing to take ownership of your life, then you're not a real man. You're just a boy playing at being a man.

So if you want to truly be a man, then it's time to stop making excuses and start taking action. It's time to face your fears and push past them. It's time to embrace discomfort and learn from your failures. It's time to set goals and hold yourself accountable for making progress towards them.

And if you're not willing to do these things, then you're not ready to be a real man. You're just another excuse-making, mediocre, cowardly boy.

So the choice is yours. Are you ready to "man up" and take ownership of your life? Or are you content to live a life of mediocrity and excuses? The answer will determine whether you're a real man or just a boy.

Now, let's talk about what it really means to take ownership of your life.

Taking ownership means accepting that you are responsible for your own success or failure. You can't blame others for your problems or expect someone else to solve them for you. You have to be willing to put in the work and take the necessary steps to achieve your goals.

It also means being accountable for your actions. You can't just make excuses or pass the buck when things go wrong. You have to own up to your mistakes and take steps to fix them. This takes courage and integrity, but it's the only way to truly grow and learn from your experiences.

One of the biggest obstacles to taking ownership is fear. Fear of failure, fear of rejection, fear of the unknown. But fear is just an illusion. It's a mental barrier that holds us back from reaching our full potential. Real men recognize their fears and push past them.

Another obstacle is comfort. It's easy to get complacent and settle for mediocrity. But real men don't settle. They strive for excellence in all areas of their lives - their careers, their relationships, their health and fitness, their personal growth.

And when they do face setbacks or failures, they don't make excuses. They take responsibility for their mistakes and use them as opportunities to learn and grow. They don't let setbacks define them - they use them as fuel to keep pushing forward.

So how do you take ownership of your life? Here are a few practical tips:

1. Set goals: Write down your goals and break them down into achievable steps. Hold yourself accountable for making progress towards those goals every day.

2. Take action: Don't wait for someone else to give you permission or motivation. Take action towards your goals every day, even if it's just a small step.

3. Face your fears: Identify your fears and push past them. Don't let fear hold you back from pursuing your dreams.

4. Embrace discomfort: Get comfortable with being uncomfortable. Growth and progress often require stepping outside of your comfort zone.

5. Learn from failures: Don't make excuses for your failures. Use them as opportunities to learn and grow. Analyze what went wrong, adjust your approach, and keep pushing forward.

Remember, being a real man is not about being perfect or infallible. It's about taking ownership of your life and striving for excellence in all areas. It's about facing your fears and pushing past them. It's about embracing discomfort and learning from your failures. It's about taking action and creating your own opportunities for success.

So if you want to be a real man in this world, it's time to stop making excuses and start taking ownership of your life. It's time to "man up" and be the best version of yourself.

G.O.A.T Rule #16 | Rise Above the Herd: How to Become a Hero Amongst the Sheep

> "
>
> *Heroes don't wait for opportunities, they create them. They don't follow trends, they set them.A hero isn't just another sheep in wolf's clothing. They're the wolf that runs with the pack but leads them to victory.*

Welcome to G.O.A.T Rule #16, where we will learn how to rise above the herd and become a hero amongst the sheep. This chapter is not for the faint of heart. It's for those who are willing to face the harsh reality of what it takes to be a real man in today's world. The truth is, being a hero is not easy. It requires hard work, dedication, and a willingness to face your fears.

Let's start by talking about setting your own trends. It's easy to follow the crowd and do what everyone else is doing, but that's not what heroes do. They have the courage to be different, to go against the grain, and to take risks. They're not afraid to fail because they know that failure is just a stepping stone on the path to success.

Take, for example, Elon Musk. He didn't follow the herd and start another software company. He went against the grain and started SpaceX, a private space exploration company. He faced numerous failures along the way, but he kept pushing forward and eventually achieved success. Now he's changing the world and inspiring others to do the same.

Another important aspect of being a hero is having a clear sense of purpose. What drives you? What are your goals and aspirations? What legacy do you want to leave behind? Heroes have a purpose that goes beyond just making money or being famous. They want to make a difference in the world and leave it a better place than they found it.

Take, for example, Malala Yousafzai. She was just a teenager when she was shot by the Taliban for speaking out about the importance of education for girls. Despite the risks, she continued to speak out and fight for what she believed in. Now she's a Nobel Prize laureate and an inspiration to millions around the world.

But being a hero also means taking responsibility for your actions and the consequences that come with them. It's easy to blame others for our failures, but that's not what heroes do. They own their mistakes and use them as an opportunity to learn and grow.

Take, for example, Michael Jordan. He's considered one of the greatest basketball players of all time, but he didn't get there by luck or talent alone. He worked tirelessly on his skills and pushed himself to be the best. He also owned his mistakes and used them to fuel his determination. He famously missed over 9,000 shots in his career, but he didn't let that stop him. He used it as motivation to work even harder and achieve even greater success.

And finally, being a hero means being a leader. It means inspiring others, creating a positive impact, and leaving a lasting legacy. Heroes don't just think about themselves, they think about how they can make a difference in the lives of others.

Take, for example, Nelson Mandela. He spent 27 years in prison for fighting against apartheid in South Africa. Despite the hardships, he never gave up his fight for equality and justice. When he was finally released, he became the first black president of South Africa and worked tirelessly to create a better future for his country and its people.

Being a hero amongst the sheep requires setting your own trends, having a clear sense of purpose, taking responsibility for your actions, and being a leader. It's not easy, but it's worth it. Don't be afraid to be different, to take risks, and to fail. Use your mistakes as an opportunity to learn and grow, and never give up on your dreams. Rise above the herd and become the hero you were meant to be.

Another important aspect of being a hero is having the courage to stand up for what you believe in, even if it means going against the crowd. Heroes are not afraid to speak their minds and defend their values, no matter how unpopular they may be. They don't conform to the opinions of others, but rather stay true to themselves and their beliefs.

To become a hero amongst the sheep, you must also cultivate a strong mindset that can withstand the challenges and obstacles that life throws your way. You must be mentally tough, resilient, and adaptable to change. Heroes don't give up easily, they keep pushing forward even when the going gets tough.

In addition, heroes are also disciplined in their actions and behaviors. They have a strong work ethic, they set goals and work diligently towards achieving them. They understand that success is not achieved overnight, but through consistent effort and hard work. They prioritize their time and focus on the things that matter, rather than wasting time on trivial pursuits.

But perhaps the most important aspect of being a hero is having a sense of humility. Heroes don't see themselves as better than others, but rather as individuals who have a responsibility to use their talents and abilities for the greater good. They acknowledge their weaknesses and seek to improve themselves, always striving to be the best version of themselves.

In conclusion, becoming a hero amongst the sheep is not an easy feat. It requires courage, purpose, discipline, mental toughness, and humility. It means standing up for what you believe in, setting your own course, and leading others towards success. But the reward is worth it - the satisfaction of knowing that you have made a positive impact in the world, and the knowledge that you have lived your life to the fullest. So go out there, rise above the herd, and become the hero you were always meant to be.

G.O.A.T Rule #17 | Stop Being a Beta: Mastering the Essential Skills for Modern Men

> **"**
>
> *In a world full of betas, it takes guts to stand up and be an alpha. But once you've tasted the thrill of victory and felt the power of your alpha skills, there's no going back to a life of mediocrity.*

As a man, you have a responsibility to be strong and capable. You can't be content with being a beta, following others and letting life pass you by. It's time to master the essential skills you need to be a real man in today's world.

First of all, you need to stop making excuses. You can't blame others for your shortcomings, you need to take ownership of your life and do what needs to be done to achieve your goals. Real men don't make excuses, they take action and get things done.

Another important skill for modern men is communication. You need to be able to articulate your thoughts and ideas clearly and confidently, both in your personal and professional life. Being able to communicate effectively will help you build stronger relationships and achieve success in all areas of your life.

Physical fitness is also an essential skill for modern men. You can't be a strong and capable man if you're not taking care of your body. You need to prioritize your health and fitness, making time for exercise and healthy eating habits. Being physically fit will not only make you feel better, but it will also give you the energy and stamina you need to tackle any challenge.

Another skill that is often overlooked is financial literacy. Real men are financially responsible and know how to manage their money effectively. You need to understand the basics of budgeting, investing, and saving so that you can build a secure financial future for yourself and your family.

Leadership is another skill that is essential for modern men. You need to be able to lead yourself and others towards success. Real men take charge, make decisions, and inspire others to follow their lead.

In addition to these skills, it's important for modern men to have a strong sense of purpose and direction. You need to know what you want out of life and work towards achieving it every day. Don't be content with mediocrity, strive for greatness and be the best version of yourself.

Now, I know that all of this may sound overwhelming, but don't worry. You don't have to master all of these skills overnight. Start small, make a plan, and work towards improving yourself every day. It's not about being perfect, it's about making progress and becoming the man you were meant to be.

If you want to stop being a beta and become a real man in today's world, you need to master the essential skills of communication, physical fitness, financial literacy, leadership, and purpose. Don't make excuses, take ownership of your life, and work towards improving yourself every day. Remember, you are capable of greatness, but it's up to you to make it a reality.

Look, I'm not here to sugarcoat things for you. Being a beta male is the absolute worst thing you can be in this world. You're weak, you're pathetic, and you're going nowhere in life. If you want to succeed, if you want to be respected, if you want to be a real man, you need to master the essential skills for modern men.

Let's start with the basics. A real man knows how to take care of himself. That means being physically fit, mentally sharp, and emotionally stable. It means taking care of your body, your mind, and your soul. It means being disciplined and consistent in your habits and routines. It means never making excuses for why you can't take care of yourself.

But being a real man is more than just taking care of yourself. It's also about being a leader. It's about having the courage to speak your mind, stand up for what you believe in, and inspire others to follow you. It's about being confident and assertive, but also humble and empathetic. It's about treating others with respect and kindness, but also holding them accountable when they fall short.

One of the most important skills for modern men is the ability to communicate effectively. You need to be able to express your thoughts and feelings clearly and concisely, whether it's in person, over the phone, or in writing. You need to be able to listen actively and empathetically, to understand the perspectives of others and to build strong relationships based on trust and mutual respect.

Another essential skill for modern men is the ability to take action. You need to be a doer, not a talker. You need to be willing to take risks, make mistakes, and learn from them. You need to be proactive, not reactive. You need to be constantly seeking new opportunities for growth and development.

And perhaps most importantly, you need to have a sense of purpose. You need to know why you're here, what you're meant to do, and what legacy you want to leave behind. You need to be driven by a sense of mission, not just by the desire for personal success or recognition.

In conclusion, if you want to stop being a beta and start being a real man, you need to master the essential skills for modern men. You need to take care of yourself, be a leader, communicate effectively, take action, and have a sense of purpose. You need to be disciplined, consistent, courageous, confident, empathetic, and proactive. You need to be the kind of man who inspires others to be their best selves, and who leaves a positive impact on the world.

G.O.A.T Rule #18 | Rise Above the Flames: How Perseverance Fuels Success in the Darkest Moments

> ❝
>
> *When life throws you into the flames, it's not the heat that defines you, it's how you rise above it that shows your true strength. Perseverance isn't just about winning the battle. It's about rising above the war and emerging victorious*

Alright, let's get real. Life isn't always sunshine and rainbows. Sometimes, it throws you into the flames and tests your mettle. But here's the thing: it's not the heat that defines you. It's how you rise above it that shows your true strength. And that's what perseverance is all about.

Perseverance isn't just about winning the battle. It's about rising above the war and emerging victorious. It's about having the mental toughness to keep going when things get tough. When you're in the midst of a trial or challenge, it can feel like the world is against you. But if you can find a way to rise above the flames, you'll come out the other side stronger and more resilient than ever before.

So, how do you rise above the flames? It starts with mindset. You need to have a mental attitude of never giving up, no matter how hard things get. You need to be willing to push through the pain, the fear, and the doubt. It won't be easy, but it will be worth it. As the saying goes, "No pain, no gain."

But perseverance isn't just about having the right mindset. It's also about having the right skills and tools. You need to have the ability to adapt and be flexible when things don't go as planned. You need to have a strong support system of people who believe in you and can help you through the tough times. And you need to have the courage to take risks and try new things, even when you're not sure if they'll work.

Another key aspect of perseverance is staying focused on your goals. When you're in the midst of a challenge, it can be easy to lose sight of what you're working towards. But you need to stay focused on your end goal and remind yourself why you started in the first place. Keep pushing forward, even if it's just one small step at a time.

Now, let's be real. Perseverance isn't always glamorous. It can be messy, it can be painful, and it can be downright ugly. But that's the thing: if you want to succeed in life, you need to be willing to get your hands dirty. You need to be willing to face the flames and rise above them, no matter how hard it may be.

So, to sum it up: perseverance is about having the right mindset, skills, and tools to rise above the flames and emerge victorious. It's about staying focused on your goals and never giving up, even when things get tough. It's about being willing to get your hands dirty and do whatever it takes to succeed.

Remember, when life throws you into the flames, it's not the heat that defines you. It's how you rise above it that shows your true strength. Rise above the flames, and you'll become unstoppable.

Perseverance is not just about winning the battle, but it's about rising above the war and emerging victorious. When life throws you into the flames, it's not the heat that defines you, it's how you rise above it that shows your true strength. The darkest moments in life can be the ones that define us, but it's how we handle those moments that truly matters. It's not about avoiding failure, it's about learning from it and using it as fuel to drive us towards success.

Take the example of Michael Jordan, one of the greatest basketball players of all time. Jordan didn't become a legend overnight. He faced countless obstacles, including being cut from his high school basketball team. But Jordan didn't let that defeat him. Instead, he used that rejection as motivation to work harder and become better.

He persevered through the setbacks and eventually became one of the most successful athletes in history.

Another example is that of J.K. Rowling, author of the Harry Potter series. Before she became a household name, Rowling faced numerous rejections from publishers who didn't believe in her writing. But she didn't let those rejections define her. She kept pushing forward, persevering through the tough times and eventually becoming one of the best-selling authors of all time.

These examples show that perseverance isn't just about being stubborn and refusing to give up. It's about having the resilience to keep pushing forward even when things get tough. It's about being able to adapt to new challenges and find ways to overcome them. Perseverance is not just about winning the battle, but it's about rising above the war and emerging victorious.

So how can you develop the power of perseverance in your own life? It starts with having a strong mindset. You need to believe in yourself and your ability to overcome obstacles. You need to be willing to take risks and face challenges head-on. You need to have the courage to fail and the strength to get back up and keep going.

Another important factor is having a support system. Surround yourself with people who believe in you and your goals. These people can help you stay motivated and provide encouragement when you face obstacles.

Perseverance is a key trait of successful people. It's not about avoiding failure; it's about using it as fuel to drive you towards success. It's about having the resilience to keep pushing forward even when things get tough. So rise above the flames, and use perseverance to fuel your success in even the darkest moments.

G.O.A.T Rule #19 | The Maverick's Way: Carving Your Own Path to Success and Leaving a Legacy

> **"**
>
> *Mavericks don't just think outside the box, they don't even acknowledge the box exists. Break free from the constraints of society and create your own reality. Mavericks are like sculptors, they shape their own destiny with every chisel and hammer blow. Don't wait for success to come to you, carve it yourself.*

Alright, let's get started on this journey of becoming a maverick and carving our own path to success and leaving a legacy. First and foremost, let's be honest with ourselves, are we content with just following the herd and doing what everyone else is doing? Or do we want to break free from the constraints of society and create our own reality?

Mavericks don't just think outside the box, they don't even acknowledge the box exists. They challenge the norms and push the boundaries to create something new and revolutionary. Are you willing to take that risk and create something that has never been done before? Or are you content with just living a mediocre life, just like everyone else?

Mavericks are like sculptors, they shape their own destiny with every chisel and hammer blow. They don't wait for someone else to shape their life, they take control and shape it themselves. They don't let their circumstances define them, they define their circumstances. They don't let failures or setbacks stop them, they use them as a stepping stone to reach greater heights.

To carve your own path to success, you need to have a clear vision of what you want to achieve. What legacy do you want to leave behind? What impact do you want to make in the world? Once you have a clear vision, the path to success becomes clearer.

But carving your own path to success isn't easy. It takes hard work, dedication, and a lot of perseverance. Mavericks don't wait for success to come to them, they carve it themselves. They don't let fear hold them back, they embrace it and use it as a fuel to drive them forward.

But being a maverick isn't just about achieving success for yourself, it's also about leaving a legacy for future generations. It's about creating something that will have a lasting impact on the world long after you're gone. Mavericks don't just live for themselves, they live for something greater than themselves.

It's time to stop waiting for permission to be great. The world doesn't give a fuck about you, so you gotta give a fuck about yourself. Be a f*cking maverick, blaze your own trail and leave a goddamn legacy behind.

But let's be real, being a maverick is not for the faint of heart. It takes balls, it takes grit, and it takes determination. You're gonna face setbacks, you're gonna fail, but that's just part of the journey. You gotta be willing to pick yourself back up and keep going.

And listen up, this is important: you gotta be willing to go against the grain. Society wants to put you in a box and label you, but you gotta break free from that shit. You gotta be willing to stand up for what you believe in, even if it means going against the f*cking crowd.

So, what are you waiting for? Are you gonna be a sheep, or are you gonna be a goddamn maverick? The choice is yours. But I'll tell you this, being a maverick is not easy, but it's worth it. The world needs more mavericks, so be the change you want to see in the world. Carve your own path to success and leave a goddamn legacy behind.

G.O.A.T Rule #20 | Survival of the Fittest: Unleashing Your Inner Leader

"

Success as a leader is reserved for those who are willing to do whatever it takes, even if it means stepping on a few toes along the way.If you're not willing to fight for your place at the top, you'll be trampled underfoot by those who are.

Listen up, son. If you want to be a real man in this world, you have to understand that success as a leader is reserved for the strong, the determined, and the unapologetic. It's a brutal world out there, and if you're not willing to fight for your place at the top, you'll be trampled underfoot by those who are.

So let me break it down for you. Being a real man means embracing your inner strength and being willing to do whatever it takes to achieve your goals. It means making tough decisions, even if they're not popular, and being willing to step on a few toes along the way. It means understanding that success is not guaranteed, and that you have to be willing to put in the hard work, to make sacrifices, and to push yourself to the limit.

But most importantly, being a real man means never giving up. You have to be willing to persevere through the tough times, to push through the pain, and to keep your eye on the prize. Because in the end, it's not about being nice, or being liked, or fitting in. It's about being a leader, and being willing to do whatever it takes to achieve your goals.

So if you want to be a real man in this era, you have to be willing to embrace your inner savage. You have to be willing to fight for what you believe in, to stand up for yourself, and to never back down from a challenge. Because in the end, that's what separates the real men from the boys.

Now, I'm not saying you have to be a heartless jerk. That's not what being a real man is about. It's about being confident in yourself, and being willing to stand up for what you believe in. It's about being a leader, not a follower. And it's about understanding that the world of leadership is a battlefield, where only the strongest and most determined will emerge victorious.

To unleash your inner leader and become a true man in this world, you have to be unapologetic about your desires and your goals. You have to be willing to take risks, to make tough decisions, and to be ruthless when necessary. You can't worry about hurting someone's feelings or making everyone happy. You have to be focused on your own success and the success of your team.

And let me tell you, son, success is not for the weak-hearted. It's for those who are willing to fight tooth and nail, to go the extra mile, and to push themselves to their limits. It's for those who are willing to make sacrifices, to work long hours, and to do whatever it takes to achieve their goals. It's for those who are unafraid to step on a few toes along the way.

So if you want to be a real man in this world, you have to be willing to embrace the harsh reality of survival of the fittest. You have to be willing to fight for your place at the top, to be unapologetically yourself, and to never back down from a challenge. It won't be easy, but I promise you, son, it will be worth it. Because in the end, there's nothing more satisfying than knowing that you fought for your success, and that you earned every single victory.

As a real man, you have to be willing to take control of your life and your destiny. You can't just sit around and wait for things to happen to you. You have to make them happen. You have to be the one who takes charge and leads the way.

And let me tell you, son, being a leader is not just about telling people what to do. It's about inspiring them, motivating them, and bringing out the best in them. It's about being the kind of person that people want to follow, because they believe in you and they believe in your vision.

So if you want to be a real man in this world, you have to be willing to be a leader. You have to be willing to take risks, to make tough decisions, and to inspire those around you to be their best selves. You have to be willing to be unapologetically yourself, and to never back down from a challenge. Because in the end, that's what real men do.

Now, I know it's not going to be easy. There will be setbacks and challenges along the way. But that's when you have to dig deep, find your inner strength, and push through the pain. Because in the end, the reward will be worth it. The reward of knowing that you fought for your success, and that you achieved your goals through hard work, determination, and a never-say-die attitude.

So go out there, son, and unleash your inner leader. Be unapologetically yourself, take control of your life, and never back down from a challenge. Because in the end, that's what it means to be a real man in this world.

G.O.A.T Rule #21 | Stop F*cking Around: How to Overcome Your Limiting Beliefs and Become the King of Your World

> **"**
>
> *Your potential is a raging inferno, but your limiting beliefs are a bucket of water. Dump that shit out and let your fire burn bright.*

Listen up, soldier. You think you've got potential? You think you've got fire inside you? Well, let me tell you something: your potential is a raging inferno, but your limiting beliefs are a bucket of water. And if you don't dump that shit out, you're gonna spend the rest of your life wondering why the fuck you're not living up to your true potential.

You wanna be the king of your world? You gotta overcome your limiting beliefs. You gotta stop making excuses and start taking action. You gotta be a warrior, not a pussy-ass victim. You gotta be willing to do whatever it takes to achieve your goals and live your best life.

So, how do you overcome your limiting beliefs? It's simple. You gotta identify them first. What are the beliefs that are holding you back? What are the thoughts that are keeping you from achieving your true potential? Write that shit down, and then tear it apart. Look at each belief and ask yourself: is this really true? Is this really holding me back? And if it's not, then dump that shit out. Let it go.

But here's the thing: it's not enough to just identify and dismantle your limiting beliefs. You gotta replace that shit with something positive. You gotta find a new belief that empowers you and motivates you. You gotta find a new thought that ignites your fire and fuels your passion. And then you gotta act on it.

Listen, I'm not gonna sugarcoat this. Overcoming your limiting beliefs is gonna be hard. It's gonna be painful. It's gonna be uncomfortable as fuck. But let me tell you something: it's worth it. Because when you overcome your limiting beliefs, you become the king of your world. You become unstoppable. You become a legend.

Here's the thing. Overcoming your limiting beliefs is not a one-time event. It's a process. It's a journey. You're gonna encounter new limiting beliefs along the way, and you're gonna have to overcome them too. It's a lifelong process of growth and development.

So, don't get complacent. Don't think that just because you've overcome some of your limiting beliefs, you're done. You're never f*cking done. You gotta keep pushing yourself, keep challenging yourself, keep growing and evolving. You gotta keep that fire burning bright.

And yeah, there are gonna be setbacks. There are gonna be times when you feel like you're backsliding. There are gonna be times when you feel like you're not making any progress. But let me tell you something: setbacks are not failures. They're opportunities. They're opportunities to learn and grow and become f*cking stronger.

So, embrace the setbacks. Embrace the challenges. Embrace the struggle. Because that's what it takes to become the king of your world. That's what it takes to achieve true success and live a life of fulfillment.

And let me tell you something else. Overcoming your limiting beliefs is not just about you. It's about the people around you too. When you overcome your limiting beliefs, you inspire others to do the same. You become a role model. You become a leader.

So, don't just do this shit for yourself. Do it for your family. Do it for your friends. Do it for your community. Be the example that others can look up to and learn from.

So, stop f*cking around. Dump that bucket of water and let your fire burn bright. Overcome your limiting beliefs and become the king of your world.

G.O.A.T Rule #22 | Warpath to Glory: Mastering the Art of War for the Modern Warrior

> *In war, you gotta be like a hawk. You gotta have eyes that can see through walls. You gotta have wings that can carry you high. And you gotta have talons that can rip through steel. The modern warrior is not just a fighter. He's a strategist. He's a leader. He's a visionary. He's the one who sees the big picture and knows how to win.*

Listen up, man. If you want to be a modern warrior, you gotta have balls of steel. You gotta have the eyes of a hawk that can see through walls and anticipate every move your enemies make. You gotta have wings that can carry you high above the fray, where you can see the big picture and make strategic decisions. And you gotta have talons that can rip through steel and crush anyone who stands in your way.

But being a modern warrior is not just about physical strength and combat skills. It's about mental toughness, discipline, and leadership. It's about having a vision for your life and the willingness to do whatever it takes to achieve your goals.

So let me tell you something, man. The world is a battlefield. It's full of challenges and obstacles that will try to hold you back and tear you down. But if you wanna be a modern warrior, you gotta face those challenges head-on and never back down.

You gotta be willing to fight for what you believe in, even if it means going against the grain and standing up to the status quo. You gotta be willing to take risks and make sacrifices, knowing that the rewards will be worth it in the end.

And most importantly, you gotta be willing to lead. You gotta be the one who sets the example for others to follow. You gotta be the one who inspires others to greatness and helps them achieve their full potential.

So let me ask you, man. Are you ready to be a modern warrior? Are you ready to step up and take on the challenges of the world? Are you ready to lead by example and inspire others to greatness?

If so, then it's time to start mastering the art of war. It's time to develop the mental and physical toughness you need to succeed. It's time to build your strategic vision and become the leader you were meant to be.

Remember, man. The world is a battlefield, and you're either a warrior or a pussy. So choose wisely, and always remember that the heart of a hawk beats within you.

Alright, let's dive deeper into what it means to be a modern warrior and how you can master the art of war.

First and foremost, you need to develop mental toughness. This means being able to withstand the pressures of life and keep going even when things get tough. One way to do this is by setting goals and then pushing yourself to achieve them, even when it seems impossible. Another way is by learning how to manage your emotions and stay calm under pressure.

But mental toughness alone won't make you a great warrior. You also need physical strength and combat skills. This means staying in shape and practicing martial arts or other forms of combat. You never know when you might need to defend yourself or others, so it's important to be prepared.

And of course, strategy is key. The art of war is all about outsmarting your opponents and winning the battle before it even begins. This means studying your enemies and knowing their weaknesses, as well as being able to anticipate their moves and plan your own accordingly.

But strategy is not just about winning battles. It's also about achieving your long-term goals and fulfilling your vision for your life. This means making strategic decisions about your career, your relationships, and your personal growth.

So how do you become a master of the art of war? Here are some suggestions:

1. Set clear goals and work towards them every day. This will help you develop the mental toughness you need to succeed.

2. Stay in shape and practice martial arts or other forms of combat. This will give you the physical strength and skills you need to defend yourself and others.

3. Study your enemies and know their weaknesses. This will help you outsmart them and win battles before they even begin.

4. Anticipate your opponents' moves and plan your own accordingly. This will help you stay one step ahead and achieve your goals more quickly.

5. Develop a strategic vision for your life and make decisions that align with it. This will help you achieve your long-term goals and fulfill your purpose.

Remember, man. The art of war is not just about winning battles. It's about becoming the best version of yourself and achieving greatness in every aspect of your life. So stay focused, stay disciplined, and never back down from a challenge.

G.O.A.T Rule #23 | F*cking Up Is Not An Option: Reaching Your Full Potential Now

> **"**
>
> *Fck fear, fck doubt, f*ck all the haters. Reaching your full potential requires you to be bold and take risks. The only thing standing between you and your full potential is yourself. Get out of your own way and make sh*t happen.*

Let me start by telling you that the road to greatness is not for the faint of heart. It's not for the weak-minded or the easily discouraged. It's for soldiers who are willing to fight for what they want, who are willing to put in the work and make sacrifices to reach their full potential.

And let me tell you something else, soldier: you can't just sit around waiting for success to come to you. You can't wait for someone else to make it happen for you. You have to take the bull by the horns and make sh*t happen. You have to be the one to create your own opportunities, to take risks, to put yourself out there and make things happen.

I know it's scary. I know it's easier said than done. But that's where the real growth and progress comes from - stepping outside your comfort zone and doing the things that scare you. Don't let fear or doubt hold you back. Don't listen to the haters and naysayers who try to bring you down.

The truth is, you're going to make mistakes along the way. You're going to f*ck up. But that's okay. That's part of the process. It's part of learning and growing. What's not okay is giving up or settling for mediocrity. You're better than that, soldier. You're meant for greatness.

So here's what you need to do: you need to dig deep and find that fire inside of you. That fire that burns bright and tells you that you're capable of achieving anything you set your mind to. You need to tap into that fire and let it fuel you. Let it drive you forward, even when things get tough.

Remember, soldier, that f*cking up is not an option. Giving up is not an option. Settling for less than your full potential is not an option. You were meant for greatness, and it's up to you to make it happen.

Let's be real, soldier. You've been playing it safe for too damn long. You're living life like a spectator instead of a player. But it's time to change that. It's time to stop sitting on the sidelines and start taking action. The only thing holding you back from reaching your full potential is your own damn self. It's time to stop making excuses and start making things happen.

So, how do you do that? How do you reach your full potential and become the best damn soldier you can be? It all starts with taking risks. I'm not talking about being reckless or stupid, but I am talking about stepping out of your comfort zone and doing things that scare you. When you take risks, you're challenging yourself and pushing yourself to be better. You're not settling for mediocrity, you're striving for greatness.

But taking risks can be scary, I get it. That's where fear and doubt come in. Fear is a natural human emotion, but it's not something that should control your life. The same goes for doubt. Doubting yourself and your abilities will only hold you back. It's time to say f*ck *fear and f*ck doubt. You're a soldier, damn it. You've been trained to handle tough situations and come out on top. Trust in yourself and your abilities.

And let's not forget about the haters. Those people who doubt you and try to bring you down. F*ck them too. You don't need their validation or approval to reach your full potential. In fact, their negativity can fuel your fire and motivate you to prove them wrong. Let their hate be the fuel that propels you forward.

Now, I'm not saying that reaching your full potential is going to be easy. It's going to take hard work and dedication. It's going to require you to be disciplined and focused. But it's worth it. The feeling of reaching your full potential and achieving your goals is indescribable. It's like nothing else in this world.

So soldier, I challenge you to take action. Take that risk, face your fears, and tell your doubts to f*ck off. *Don't let anyone or anything hold you back from reaching your full potential. It's time to unleash the beast within and make sh*t happen.*

G.O.A.T Rule #24 | The Freedom Manifesto: Rejecting Society's Rules and Living on Your Own Terms

> **"**
>
> *Society wants to control you like a puppet, but real men cut the strings and dance to their own beat. Life is too short to live by someone else's rules. Take charge and write your own story*

Today, we're going to talk about true freedom - the kind that comes from living life on your own terms. Society wants to control us, mold us into their image, and dictate how we should live our lives. But real men reject those strings and cut them loose, dancing to their own beat and living life on their own terms.

We all have a unique story to write in this life, and it's up to us to decide what that story looks like. Are you going to let society dictate your story, or are you going to take charge and write your own? It's time to stop being a puppet and start being the puppet master.

One of the biggest obstacles to living life on your own terms is fear. Fear of the unknown, fear of failure, fear of judgment. But fear is nothing more than a mental barrier that we create for ourselves. We have the power to overcome it and achieve true freedom. It starts with recognizing the fear, acknowledging it, and then taking action in spite of it.

Another obstacle is conformity. Society wants us to conform to their standards, but real men don't conform. We don't settle for mediocrity or follow the herd. We blaze our own trail and stand out from the crowd. It takes courage and confidence to go against the grain, but it's worth it.

Living life on your own terms also means taking responsibility for your own happiness. It's not society's job to make us happy - that's our job. We have the power to choose our own path and create the life we want. Happiness is a choice, and it's up to us to make that choice.

So, soldier, I urge you to reject society's rules and live life on your own terms. Cut the strings, dance to your own beat, and write your own story. Don't let fear or conformity hold you back from achieving true freedom. Take responsibility for your own happiness and create the life you want. Remember, you are the puppet master, not the puppet.

It's time to stop letting society dictate how you should live your life. You need to break free from the chains of social conformity and start living on your own terms. Society wants you to believe that conformity is the only way to succeed in life, but that's complete bullshit.

The truth is that conformity is for the weak. Real men reject the status quo and chart their own path in life. They don't wait for someone else to give them permission to succeed. They take charge and make their own way in the world.

But the road to true freedom is not an easy one. It requires courage, determination, and a willingness to face your fears head-on. You will be criticized, mocked, and ridiculed by those who are too afraid to step out of their comfort zone. But if you stay true to yourself and keep pushing forward, you will eventually break through the barriers that have been holding you back.

The key to living life on your own terms is to focus on what truly matters to you. Don't let other people's opinions and expectations determine your path in life. You need to be true to yourself and follow your passions, even if it means going against the grain.

Remember, soldier, the road to true freedom is not a smooth one. You will encounter obstacles and setbacks along the way. But if you stay true to yourself and keep pushing forward, you will eventually reach your destination.

In the end, the only person who can truly control your life is you. You have the power to create your own destiny and live life on your own terms. So go out there and grab life by the balls. Reject society's rules and start living life on your own terms. The world is waiting for you, soldier.

Let's talk about what it means to live life on your own terms. It means being the master of your own destiny, and not letting anyone else dictate how you should live your life. It means taking responsibility for your own happiness and well-being, and not relying on others to provide it for you.

Living life on your own terms requires a certain level of confidence and courage. It means being willing to take risks and make bold decisions, even if they are not popular or conventional. It also means being comfortable with uncertainty and ambiguity, and not needing to have everything figured out in advance.

The key to living life on your own terms is to be clear about what you truly value and what you want to achieve in life. This requires introspection and self-reflection, as well as the courage to pursue your dreams and goals, even if they seem impossible or unlikely.

Of course, living life on your own terms is not always easy. There will be obstacles and challenges along the way, and you may face resistance and criticism from others who don't understand or support your choices. But true freedom comes from being able to overcome these obstacles and stay true to yourself and your values, even in the face of adversity.

So, my advice to you, soldier, is this: don't be afraid to challenge the status quo and live life on your own terms. It may not always be easy or comfortable, but it is the only way to truly achieve lasting happiness and fulfillment. Remember, the only person who can truly control your life is you.

G.O.A.T Rule #25 | Crushing the Status Quo: Building the Life You Want, Not What Society Tells You to Have

> *If you want to live like a king, you gotta stop thinking like a peasant. Stop waiting for permission to live your dream life. Give yourself permission and start making it happen.*

Alright, soldier. Let's talk about crushing the status quo and building the life you really want. It's time to stop being a little bitch and start taking control of your life.

You know what society wants for you? They want you to be a good little worker bee, toiling away for 40+ hours a week just to make someone else rich. They want you to be content with a mediocre existence, never striving for anything better. But you're better than that, aren't you? You're a warrior, a fighter, a goddamn king. You deserve to live life on your own terms.

So what's holding you back? Fear? Doubt? Bullshit excuses? Cut that shit out. Stop waiting for permission to live the life you want. Give yourself permission to be great, to be f*cking unstoppable. Stop thinking like a peasant and start thinking like a king.

You want to live like a king? Then start acting like one. Stop settling for crumbs and start demanding the whole damn cake. It's time to stop playing small and start playing to win.

But here's the thing, soldier. Building the life you want isn't easy. It takes work. It takes sacrifice. It takes taking risks and stepping out of your comfort zone. It takes crushing the status quo and doing things differently than everyone else.

But it's worth it. Oh, is it worth it. Because living your dream life is f*cking amazing. It's waking up every day with purpose and passion. It's doing work that you love and that makes a difference. It's having the time and freedom to do the things you enjoy with the people you love.

So stop waiting for the stars to align and start making shit happen. Take action towards your goals every damn day. Surround yourself with people who support and encourage you. And most importantly, believe in yourself and your ability to create the life you want.

Remember, soldier, you only have one life to live. Don't waste it living someone else's dream. Build the life you want and live it with everything you've got.

Don't let the fear of failure hold you back. Failure is a part of the journey towards success. Embrace it and use it as fuel to drive you forward. And don't let the opinions of others dictate your choices. You know what you want and what you're capable of, so go out there and make it happen.

One thing that's important to remember is that building the life you want isn't easy. It requires hard work, dedication, and perseverance. You're going to face obstacles and challenges along the way, but that's all part of the process. Don't let setbacks discourage you. Keep pushing forward and stay focused on your goals.

Another important factor is to be mindful of the company you keep. Surround yourself with people who support your dreams and encourage you to be your best self. Stay away from those who try to bring you down or hold you back. You don't need that negativity in your life.

Finally, don't forget to enjoy the journey. Building the life you want is not just about reaching the end goal, it's about the experiences and growth that come with it. Take time to appreciate the small victories and milestones along the way. Celebrate your progress and remember to have fun.

Crushing the status quo and building the life you want is possible, but it requires hard work, dedication, and a willingness to go against the norm. Don't let fear or the opinions of others hold you back. Embrace failure and setbacks as part of the journey towards success. Surround yourself with positive and supportive people, and remember to enjoy the process. With these tools, you can create the life of your dreams and live on your own terms.

I want to remind you that you have the power to create the life you want. You don't have to settle for a mediocre existence dictated by society's rules and expectations. You can break free from the chains that bind you and start living on your own terms.

But I must be brutally honest with you: it won't be easy. It will take hard work, determination, and a willingness to embrace discomfort and uncertainty. You will face obstacles, setbacks, and criticism. You will have to make sacrifices and take risks. But if you stay focused on your vision, trust in yourself, and keep pushing forward, you will reach your goals.

Remember, living the life of your dreams is not just about achieving material success or accumulating wealth. It's about finding fulfillment, happiness, and meaning in your life. It's about living with purpose and intention, and making a positive impact on the world around you.

So don't let fear or self-doubt hold you back. Don't let society's expectations define your life. Take control of your destiny and create the life you want. Be bold, be courageous, and be true to yourself.

In the words of the Top G, "You only live once, but if you do it right, once is enough." So go out there and make it count. Crush the status quo, build the life you want, and live your dream.

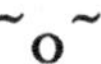

Congratulations, soldier. You've made it to the end of this book. You've learned the G.O.A.T rules, absorbed the harsh realities, and hopefully, found the motivation to become a real man in this era. But don't let this be the end. The real challenge begins now. It's time to put everything you've learned into action. It's time to take charge of your life, reject mediocrity, overcome limiting beliefs, and build the life you truly desire. Remember, you have the potential to be a king, but it won't happen by chance. You must make it happen. So go out there, be bold, take risks, and never settle for less than you deserve.

More Books Coming! Time to re-build men to become Top G's